Your Guide in
Nutrition & Healthy Living

Your Guide in Nutrition & Healthy Living

Food Wisdom Series

By Miriam Moras

Your Guide in Nutrition & Healthy Living

Third edition November 2024
Published by Broccoli People
ISBN: 978-84-09-64247-2

This book aims to raise awareness and educate about health, motivating readers to educate themselves on important topics and encouraging support of environmentally friendly practices that enhance overall well-being.

It does not provide medical recommendations to treat specific conditions and should not be used as a substitute for medical advice. Readers should consult with their doctor regarding any health-related matters.

broccolipeople@gmail.com
www.broccolipeople.com

About Broccoli People

Broccoli People's books aim to provide accessible and practical information on health and nutrition. In today's world, the amount of information and controversies can be confusing and overwhelming. Therefore, the objective here is to simplify these topics. The author, Miriam Moras, a health coach specialised in nutrition, created this series with the intention to offer simple and accessible guides emphasising the holistic nature of health and well-being.

You won't find the latest trendy diets or new products, but rather guidelines to be adapted for each person. However, the fields of nutrition and well-being are constantly evolving, and there is always much left to be discovered. As a result, there have already been several revisions to keep the books up-to-date.

Afterward, if you are interested and want to explore specific topics further, you can continue your journey of learning and exploring life as a never ending process.

As Marie Curie said,
"Nothing is to be feared, only to be understood."

"Your Guide in Nutrition & Healthy Living"

Take ownership of your health,
be more conscious about your choices,
and more mindful of your actions.

Learn the principles of nutrition,
understand more about holistic living,
realise the magic nature of your body,
and start paying attention to it.

You will get some practical tools,
find out about the latest trends,
how to make good choices,
and to adapt it to your conditions.

Healthier and happier go together
and you can now be proactive in working on both;
nobody else can do it for you.

Contents

1. Happiness

The happiness-health connection

Happiness is an interesting concept. It depends on our conceptual filters of reality, perception, and interpretation. It is complicated, but let's start talking about what the body needs to experience physical harmony and mental clarity.

We know that there is a direct connection between physical and emotional states. The brain and nervous system have specific physical needs, which, if not met, will have mental and emotional consequences. They can trigger sensations followed by reactions and emotions, affecting your mood and experience of life. Have you ever had back pain and ended up grumpy and arguing with everyone? Or nutritional deficiencies that led to low energy and mood swings?

Happiness is related to connection, fun, and vitality, while unhappiness is related to stress, worries, unexpressed emotions, and decay. The other way is also true, happiness makes you healthier, while unhappiness can lead to physical problems. In the end, neither happiness without health, nor health without joy, may be very healthy.

In modern times when we are more aware of the environmental impact of our behaviour, we also try to find new ways to base our happiness and well-being that are more in harmony with the rest of life —not at the cost of it. And that applies to evolving modern diets.

Changing oneself is the first step within your control, and note that personal evolution and happiness have a ripple effect and positively impact others—they are both easily spread! Besides the world that you carry inside, you also depend on the one outside, and your choices affect both. You are not an isolated entity.

2. Principles of Nutrition

2.1. What you and your food are made of

Your body and food are made of the same chemical elements found in nature. These elements are rearranged in different combinations to form various life forms, but we are all made of the same thing.

Your body is an ensemble of parts. The tiniest living units in you are called cells, which come together according to their type and function to form tissues, then organs, and finally systems. Your body is constantly changing and renewing itself as cells are replaced. And if this process doesn't occur correctly, it can lead to health issues.

You get two types of molecules from food: macronutrients and micronutrients. Macronutrients include proteins, carbohydrates, fats, and water, which are present in large quantities. Micronutrients, on the other hand, are present in smaller doses and include minerals, vitamins, and phytonutrients. Phytonutrients are lesser-known components found in plants that have plenty of health benefits..

Proteins are composed of smaller particles called amino acids, fats are composed of fatty acids, and carbohydrates are composed of simple sugars. These macronutrients are mainly used to produce energy, build the body, and regenerate each part. On the other hand, micronutrients facilitate chemical reactions and bodily functions, similar to how an igniter starts a fire.

Every cell requires specific nutrients to carry out its functions and support the overall functioning of the body. Therefore, nutrient deficiencies can create imbalances and result in health issues. The body is an ensemble of parts, each with its own specific functions and needs to be met for the whole body to work in harmony.

2.2. How your body digests food

Digestion involves breaking down food into smaller pieces mainly through the movement of the digestive tract. This is followed by the breakdown of complex molecules into simpler ones by specific enzymes, and eventually, the absorption of nutrients. The digestive tract is over 7.5 meters long, and the entire process of food digestion can take anywhere from 18 to 72 hours. If this process takes longer, it could be harmful for your body and could indicate underlying health issues as the root cause.

The majority of digestion actually takes place in the small intestine, not in the stomach. Initially, the pancreas secretes its juices, while the gallbladder secretes bile produced by the liver to help digestion. Most nutrients are then absorbed through the wall of the small intestine, and the rest continues into the large intestine.

Once nutrients are absorbed, they pass to the liver, which act like a filter, and later into the bloodstream. The liver determines what enter the bloodstream and removes potential toxins.

Water is absorbed in the big intestine, where a large amounts and varieties of bacteria live and transform undigested food into essential nutrients for the body. They feed themselves on it, and in a symbiotic relationship, they turn some undigested nutrients into essential components for the body to use. For example, they transform fibre into certain essential fats.

Additionally, the gut has its own nervous system that controls intestinal processes and movements, producing neurotransmitters such as serotonin and dopamine, leading to its nickname as "the second brain."

Your body has an equilibrium that it will always try to maintain because that's where conditions are the best for its functioning, and it will do anything to return to that equilibrium. This steady state of internal conditions is called homeostasis.

It shows how the perfect state can only be defined in balance, and nature will always strive to find that equilibrium by itself, regardless of what we do. The natural movement of everything is to reach those states, which also happens inside us, following a flow toward harmony.

In practice, this means that whatever you do or eat that pushes you beyond those required levels will create an imbalance. The body will detect and try to compensate for it by maintaining homeostasis at any expense.

For example, if the body temperature is too high, sweating will cool it down, and shivering will raise it if it is too low. If the concentration of calcium circulating through the bloodstream drops below optimal levels, the body will take it from the bones to raise it. Or, if the glucose levels are too high, the pancreas will release insulin to lower it. And the exact mechanism happens for other levels of components like sodium, potassium, and blood pressure.

Anything that disturbs the required equilibrium makes the body react, which will have effects elsewhere, similar to a ripple effect.

All of this shows that the body is smart enough to regulate and heal when conditions change. The real solutions in nature rely on finding and consistently maintaining that perfect balance.

2.4. You are what you absorb

You are what you digest, absorb, and transfer into your cells. It is not only about what you eat but what finally reaches your cells—the tiniest living units that make up your body.

Intolerances, allergies, leaky gut, the permeability of cell membranes, stress, and other conditions can reduce your capacity to absorb those nutrients properly. However, you can prevent all this with the diet and lifestyle you adopt. The guidelines in this book will help you with that.

2.5. Gut health

The human body has trillions of microorganisms from thousands of varieties that are non-human cells, which means that they have different DNA from yours. They are the human microbiota and play essential roles in your health. Their number and types vary for each person, and those differences can impact their health or predisposition to develop certain conditions.

Concretely, gut microbiota or gut flora refers to microorganisms living in the digestive tract with a symbiotic relationship with your body. They help defend against harmful organisms, with digestion and absorption of some nutrients, producing specific vitamins and fats, and even sending signals to the brain through the gut-brain axis.

The quantity and diversity of gut bacteria depend on your diet, lifestyle, and early childhood. Imbalances are associated with many modern health issues, such as immune and inflammatory conditions, food intolerances, obesity, skin problems, chronic fatigue, IBS, autism, and depression. It is a fascinating new field that shows us the essential roles of gut health in our physical and mental well-being.

Macronutrients are the nutrients in food in large quantities, and as previously explained, your body uses them to produce energy and build itself up. Each person has different requirements, and your body, gender, and lifestyle dictate the quantities and proportions you need them.

Proteins

Proteins are the building blocks that form part of every cell and make your body's muscles and other structures. They are involved in essential body functions like helping to recover and build muscle, replacing cells, forming neurotransmitters and hormones, balancing fluids, and boosting the immune system. They are composed of amino acids, nine of which are essential because the body can't produce them and must get them from food. Foods containing all the essential nine are called complete or good-quality protein sources.

Carbohydrates

Carbohydrates or carbs are the first sources of energy for your body. The amount the body can store is small, called glycogen stores, only in the liver and muscles. However, the body can also get energy from all the other macronutrients, like fats and protein. It depends on how fast the energy is needed, your diet, and the glycogen stores.

In addition, carbs play other important roles; therefore, diets that restrict them are advisable for short periods or with periodic breaks to avoid disrupting those different functions.

Fats are stored in the most significant amounts for energy use and play essential roles in the brain, nervous system, immunity, and hormonal balance. As already mentioned, the body needs all nutrients in the proper proportions, including fats.

The ratio between different types of fats in modern society is usually out of balance, often with deficiencies in Omega 3 and unsaturated fats while excessive Omega 6 and saturated fats.

2.7. Fats

Fats are a type of macronutrient made of smaller particles called fatty acids, the main components of the brain and the highest energy source.

They used to be blamed for the increasing obesity in the modern world. However, obesity was mainly due to other factors, like sedentary lifestyles, overconsumption of ultra-processed foods, excessive sugars, sleep deprivation, and stress. Ultra-processed foods usually contain too much white sugar, saturated fats, and other additives that give them an addictive effect, making it too easy to overeat them.

Fats are essential, but not all fats are created equal. While all types of fats are necessary, an imbalance in their consumption can lead to health issues. For instance, many processed foods contain saturated fats in ratios 18–20 times higher than other fats, or they may include trans fats, which are the only type of fat that is not needed and should be avoided according to recommendations.

Omega 3 sources: oily fish (e.g., salmon, sardines, mackerel, and tuna), flaxseeds, walnuts, and chia seeds.

Omega 6 sources: most vegetable oils (especially safflower, soybeans, corn, and sunflower oils), processed products with these oils, fast foods, and sunflower seeds.

Omega 3 is a fat often lacking in modern diets, and we can't overemphasise its importance. It is essential for the brain, nervous, and immune systems. Increasing its intake can be very beneficial in cases of inflammation, auto-immune diseases, bone problems, mood swings, poor concentration, and preventing degenerative conditions like Parkinson's and Alzheimer's.

Omega 6 has the opposite effect of Omega 3. The body needs both types of fats in the right balance, but nowadays Omega 6 is typically consumed in much higher quantities. As a result, it is advisable to lower the intake of Omega 6 while increasing Omega 3 in your diet. Moreover, note that Omega 3 from animal sources is better absorbed and utilised by the body than from plant sources or supplements.

2.9. Micronutrients

Micronutrients are chemicals needed in small doses. They act as the ignitors or catalysts of reactions that would not occur otherwise. For example, most B vitamins facilitate energy production, vitamin D helps calcium absorption, and vitamin C assists in iron absorption. Consequently, their deficiencies would disrupt many bodily functions and reactions. Below is an overview of the main micronutrients.

Calcium: about 99% of the calcium is in your bones and teeth structure; however, it also plays important roles in blood clotting, helping muscles to contract, and regulating heart rhythms and nerve functions. Sources are dairy, almonds, beans, broccoli, spinach, kale, firm tofu, sardines, and fortified foods.

Magnesium: more than 300 biochemical reactions in the body depend on magnesium. It participates in nerve and muscle functions, supports the immune system and wound healing, keeps the heartbeat steady, helps bones remain strong, and is part of blood sugar level regulation. Food sources are whole grains, pumpkin seeds, almonds, cashews, peanuts, sesame seeds, beans, spinach, milk, cocoa, molasses, salmon, okra, bananas, apples, and avocados.

Iron: participates in synthesising hemoglobin and energy production, supports the immune system, and forms part of enzymes. Food sources are beef, oysters, molasses, lentils, beans, chickpeas, kidney beans, spinach, eggs, soybeans, pumpkin seeds, sesame seeds, cashews, and figs.

Vitamin D: is essential for bone health and the immune system. For example, the body requires adequate levels of vitamin D to absorb and use calcium. It is primarily synthesised from direct exposure to sunlight, and only a few foods are sources of vitamin D, such as oily fish, egg yolks, and fortified foods.

Fluoride: is an important mineral to maintain strong teeth. Food sources are fish bones, water, tea, and some poultry.

Choline: is essential for brain health and early brain development in pregnancy. Sources are eggs, beef, chicken, and soybeans.

B vitamins: are absolutely essential for brain and nervous system health and energy production. Food sources are fish, meat, grains, spinach, mushrooms, broccoli, avocados, and nuts.

Vitamin C: has essential roles in supporting the immune system and producing certain neurotransmitters. It also acts as an antioxidant and is required for iron absorption. Sources are citrus, guava, berries, broccoli, pepper, and spinach.

Potassium: is an electrolyte that helps maintain normal levels of fluid inside cells and participates in energy production. Sources are bananas, avocados, raisins, almonds, beans, lentils, potatoes, coconut water, broccoli, and dairy.

Sodium: is the counteract of potassium and maintains normal fluid levels inside cells. It also helps regulate blood pressure, nerve impulses, muscle contractions, and mineral balance.

Copper: the body needs copper for a healthy brain, immune and nervous systems, and functions such as energy production. Food sources are shellfish, seeds, nuts, organ meats, and whole grains.

Phosphorus: plays many roles and is crucial for bones, teeth, cell membranes, and energy production. Food sources are fish, meat, legumes, grains, eggs, nuts, seeds, bananas, and dairy.

Vitamin A: vision, growth, cell division, reproduction, and immunity need vitamin A. Sources: oily fish, liver, egg yolks, sweet potato, kale, and carrots.

Vitamin E: an antioxidant that participates in nerve functions and the immune system. Sources are olives, nuts, avocados, carrots, spinach, and grains.

2.10. B vitamins

There are eight vitamins in this group, and they are related to energy production, brain and nervous system health, and supporting your immunity. B vitamins are essential for brain development during childhood and for maintaining cognitive functions and preventing neurological deterioration afterward. In some cases, deficiencies for long periods can be the underlying cause of emotional dysfunctions such as irritability, nervousness, sleeplessness, depression, weakness, or cognitive decline.

The most popular ones are B9 or folic acid, especially during pregnancy, and B12, which you can read more about below. Some food sources of B9 are dark green leafy veggies, beans, peanuts, berries, whole grains, seafood, eggs, liver, and fortified foods.

2.11. B12

B12, or cobalamin, is naturally found in animal foods, but you can also find it added to foods or supplements nowadays. B12 is needed to form red blood cells and DNA and is a crucial player in the function and development of brain and nerve cells.

The body has stores that can last for a certain time when not consumed in the diet. Deficiencies can be due to not consuming animal products or supplements, or because of digestive problems that prevent your body from absorbing nutrients. Initial symptoms can be a tingling sensation in the hands or feet, excessive weakness, fatigue, or confusion. Food sources include egg yolks, all dairy products, fish (especially oily fish), seafood, meat, fortified yeast, and fortified foods.

However, how much the body can absorb iron depends on several factors. For example, vitamin C is needed to absorb iron, while certain nutrients, such as calcium, tea, and coffee, can reduce the absorption. Also, the body can absorb less iron from plant-based sources than from animal sources.

Therefore, plant-based diets need to pay attention to their iron levels and may need supplementation. Iron and calcium supplements should be taken at different times of the day. In some cases, iron blood infusion may be necessary. Some food sources of iron are beef, liver, mussels, chickpeas, lentils, cacao, pumpkin seeds, spinach, and figs.

2.13. Magnesium

Magnesium is one of the minerals present in more reactions in the body. It helps to maintain normal nerve and muscle function and is essential for recovery after intense exercise. It also helps to have better quality sleep, supports the immune system, keeps the heartbeat steady, helps bones remain strong, and aids in producing energy and protein.

Therefore, athletes and people with sleeping troubles often take magnesium supplementation to release symptoms or have better physical performance and recovery. Magnesium can be taken orally with tablets or through the skin with a spray or a bath of Epsom salts. However, for those without deficiencies, the recommendation is to boost its level through the skin, as this method is unlikely to cause any side effects or other concerns. Additionally, it's important to include more food sources, such as dairy, broccoli, green leafy vegetables, almonds, beans, tofu, fish with bones, and fortified foods.

2.14. Calcium

Calcium is the most abundant mineral in the body. Besides being related to bone health, it also has roles in nerve functions, blood clotting, muscle contractions, heartbeat regulation, and fluid balance within cells. We must have it present in our diet to preserve bone structure. When there are low calcium levels in the blood, the body eventually takes it from the bones, leading to possible future conditions if this imbalanced situation is maintained in the long term. This is an important aspect to consider during long periods of fasting while seeking other potential benefits.

Calcium works with vitamin D, which enhances calcium absorption, and vitamin K, which helps accumulate calcium in bones and teeth. Some good sources of calcium are yogurt, kefir, sesame seeds or tahini, firm tofu, almonds, green leaves, sardines, and white beans.

2.15. Bone health

As discussed in this section, several minerals and vitamins are essential in bone health. These include calcium, magnesium, vitamin D, and vitamin K, and they are all interconnected. That means that a deficiency in one may affect the absorption of another, and when there are nutrient deficiencies, there are usually a few. Everything is interconnected in the body. Moreover, the body can store calcium in the bones up to around 30s, and afterward will maintain or decline it.

Women need to pay attention to this, especially after around age 35, when their estrogen levels begin to decrease slightly. Estrogen levels peak in every menstrual cycle and are crucial for maintaining strong bones. Therefore, regular and healthy cycles are vital for women's bone health.

means that more than half of our bodies consist of this element. We need to consume water regularly because we lose it even without moving, just by breathing. We can survive for longer periods without food than we can without water.

Water is needed to dissolve nutrients and bring them to the cells. It also helps to regulate body temperature and serves as the medium for many bodily reactions. Water is everywhere, inside and outside your cells, in every tissue and structure—even in the bones, which are 30% water. Therefore, get the habit of sipping water through the day to avoid thirst, and to increase your intake in hot and tropical climates. Note that common signs of dehydration can be feeling tired or even a bit hungry. In such cases, you don't need food but to drink.

Nowadays, the issue is the quality of the water. It can be contaminated with chemicals since pollutants and pesticides can reach water sources. Additionally, water may also be depleted of minerals. In other words, we depend on water as an essential natural resource. You can take it as another reason to minimise pollution and reduce unnecessary consumption, thereby contributing to the cleanliness of the earth, including its waters.

2.17. Phytonutrients

Phytonutrients, also known as phytochemicals, are chemicals produced by plants which they use to stay healthy and safe. These compounds can also be very beneficial for humans in the long term, helping to preserve health and prevent disease, but they are not essential for our survival.

Some of those benefits for humans are antioxidant and anti-inflammatory activities. They may also enhance immunity, repair DNA damage from toxins exposure, and support detoxification processes.

Foods rich in phytonutrients include colourful fruits and vegetables, legumes, nuts, tea, whole grains, and many spices. Many phytonutrients give their pigments to plants with deep or bright colours. Therefore, the recommendation is to add a greater variety of colours of vegetables and fruits. Some examples are dark greens, berries, turmeric, onions, and garlic.

2.18. Think in nutrients, not in calories

All the nutrients mentioned previously are essential for the body to reach balance and carry out its functions. While the body needs calories to stay alive, it also requires other micronutrients. If your diet mainly consists of foods that are high in calories but low in nutritional value, you may be at risk of developing nutrient deficiencies, obesity, and other health problems. Paradoxically, malnutrition and being overweight often happen simultaneously in modern society.

Diseases often start like this, with imbalances in your diet, lifestyle, or spirituality that are ignored until the consequences become tangible. Everything in the body is interconnected; deficiencies of any of them would cause imbalances somewhere else, as in a cascade. The same applies to nutrient deficiencies.

Prioritise quality food, which is nutrient-dense food with minimal artificial additives. You don't need to count calories; that is a small part of the equation of what your body needs. Reduce ultra-processed foods and make nutrient-dense foods your primary choice.

3. Practical Guidelines

3.1. The compound effect of small habits

The habits you consistently repeat over the long term and the foods you regularly eat in your daily life have the most impact on your body. Quick diets or fast solutions are often driven by business and marketing and can be a way to maintain the same unhealthy patterns without feeling too guilty about it – essentially masking a problem so it appears different, but still remains the same underneath.

For effective results, it's not necessary to be perfect all the time or to follow every recommendation you come across, which can be overwhelming and confusing. What's more important is to be consistent in the long term rather than striving for perfection. This principle applies to all aspects of life, including changes in your food choices and lifestyle.

You can follow the "80/20" rule, which suggests that you can make progress and reap the benefits of a healthy lifestyle by following its guidelines 80% of the time, and allowing yourself to indulge 20% of the time without guilt. This gradual approach helps in establishing new habits and laying the foundations for long-term positive changes.

Start making small positive changes from wherever you are at the present moment. Keep moving forward with small improvements and trust the process without over-focusing on big end goals, as they can overshadow your effort and progress. Think of habits as the compound interest of self-improvement and the path to significant transformations resulting from many small, regular, wise steps. These small habits have a compound effect that multiplies as you repeat them.

3.2. More unprocessed and natural foods

Food processing is the whole spectrum of steps to make a final product, from ultra-processed packaged snack foods to minimally processed items like hummus or guacamole. As a result, there are various categories of processed foods, and it's important to make wise choices by primarily obtaining calories from whole, natural foods.

Whole foods have a higher nutrient density, meaning they contain more vitamins, minerals, and fibre that are all essential for your well-being. The modern diet paradox is the simultaneous presence of both nutrient deficiencies and obesity due to the low nutritional quality and low cost of ultra-processed foods.

Focus on replacing foods with healthier alternatives and adding more nutritious foods to your diet instead of restricting yourself. Check nutritional labels to understand what you're consuming. If a product has a long list of ingredients that you don't recognise and high levels of sugars and saturated fats, it is probably better to leave it on the shelf.

3.3. Balanced meals and the shopping list

Your nutritional needs depend on your body type, gender, and lifestyle. However, in practice, there are easy and intuitive ways to simplify it while you start paying more attention to what your body signals. Tuning into your body may take some time if you are new to it. Start by eating slowly!

Protein: 1-2 palm

Carbohydrates: 1-2 fist

Good fat: 1-2 thumb

Vegetables: 1-2 cupped hand

You can use the guidelines on the previous page that take hands-size portions as a reference. Note that women would usually need one measure and men two measures. Alternatively, you can fill up half of your plate with vegetables, one quarter with protein, and another quarter with carbohydrates, and boost it with a portion of healthy fats. The next step is to stock your pantry with the following shopping list.

Shopping list

Choose different foods from each group, alternate them, put variety and colours, and extend the list with regional and local products from your area.

Vegetables -> Broccoli, spinach, kale, lettuce, rocket, sunflower sprouts, morning glory, watercress, courgette, celery, pumpkin, cauliflower, carrots, Brussels sprouts, green beans, and beetroot.

Protein -> Fish, meat, eggs, cheese, yogurt, protein powders, and vegetarian/vegan source in section 4.2.

Carbohydrates -> Lentils, chickpeas, beans, brown rice, amaranth, polenta, quinoa, corn, sweet potato, potato, cassava, oats, sourdough bread, pasta, and rice noodles.

Fats-> Healthy oils: extra virgin olive oil, sesame, walnut, avocado, flaxseeds. Others: avocados, nuts (e.g. Brazil nuts, almonds, walnuts, hazelnuts, or macadamia), and all seeds (e.g. pumpkin, sesame, or chia).

Fruits -> Apples, berries, guavas, oranges, pears, peaches, papaya, grapefruit, pineapple, bananas, figs, durian, and watermelon.

Fermented foods -> Yoghurt, kefir, sauerkraut, kimchi, and miso.

3.4. Meal timing

Experts previously suggested that eating smaller quantities more frequently would help regulate blood sugar levels and fuel the body in a stable way. However, recent research has shown that this is not necessarily true, and eating too frequently can have the opposite effect that was once considered. There has also been much research on the possible benefits of controlled fasting to help reduce insulin levels, regulate blood sugar, and manage conditions like type 2 diabetes. The truth is that there is not one way that fits all, and it depends on each person and the stage of life they're in. It's not the same for a teenager, a woman in her thirties, or a man in his fifties.

The general guidelines are three balanced meals with a regular eating window, which means starting and finishing eating at a regular time every day. This habit can help regulate your circadian rhythm, which is an internal process that responds to the environment and regulates the sleep-wake cycle and your body functions and repeats every 24 hours.

Fasting has been widely studied and discussed due to its health benefits. The most popular schedule is intermittent fasting, which involves a fasting window of 12 to 16 hours at night. Many studies have shown the healing and recovery benefits of these practices, but it also depends on the individual, lifestyle, and gender.

For example, most studies have focused on men without considering the cyclical changes in women. Women are generally more sensitive to longer fasts, especially during the second part of the cycle and their period. As a result, it is recommended for women to keep from 8 to 12 hours. Be realistic about your lifestyle and situation, and make changes as simple as possible. If they are simple to put in practice, you are more likely to adopt them in the long term.

Circadian rhythm is a natural, internal process that regulates the sleep-wake cycle and repeats roughly every 24 hours, regulated mainly by light and dark.

It is essential for overall health and regulating body functions, such as detoxification and repair during sleep, as well as maintaining hormonal balances. This rhythm changes through stages in life, which is why teens are more likely to not feel tired until later in the night than adults, even though they still require more hours of sleep.

Disruption of the circadian rhythm can cause short and long-term health conditions, such as excessive tiredness, depression, poor concentration, blood sugar level imbalances, gastrointestinal conditions, obesity, and cardiovascular problems.

Regularity in your schedule is important to keep a healthy circadian rhythm. This includes consistently waking up and going to bed at similar times during the whole week, as well as the starting and finishing meals times. Try to adhere to a similar eating window and allow enough overnight fasting hours so that the body can complete all repair processes required. The right amount of fasting hours depends on the person, age, and gender, typically ranging from 8 to 16 hours.

Having morning sunlight exposure directly to the eyes without sunglasses is also important. In addition, try to avoid blue light in the evening to have healthy melatonin levels at the right time. Manage your stress levels by reducing or skipping caffeine and alcohol some hours before bedtime. And make sure to engage in regular physical activity, such as taking daily walks in the sunlight or using the stairs instead of the lift.

3.6. The healing power of sleeping

Sleep is crucial for our well-being as it allows the body and mind to repair and recover. Two phases alternate in several night cycles: NREM (non-rapid eye movement) and REM (rapid eye movement). During NREM, the body undergoes deep sleep, repairing and regenerating itself, strengthening the immune system, and consolidating memories and information. Following NREM, REM is the dreaming stage that plays essential roles in integrating events, enhancing creativity, emotional processing, healthy brain development, and memory.

The amount of sleep each person needs can range from 7 to 9. However, some individuals claim they can function well with less sleep than that, but the reality is that most sleep-deprived people are unaware of it and of the impact of their well-being. You can find some practical guidelines to improve your sleep routine in the previous section, "Circadian Rhythm."

3.7. Regulating blood sugar levels

Blood sugar, also known as glucose, is the primary energy source for your body. It fluctuates throughout the day and the more consistent and stable they are, the better your energy and mood will be.

Refined carbs, sugars, lack of fibre, sedentarism, stress, and sleep deprivation are some of the factors that can cause rapid glucose fluctuations, making you feel tired and sleepy when blood sugar drops fast. Spiky and erratic blood sugar levels with highs and lows, or constantly high, is a common pattern of modern lifestyles that can lead to health conditions such as brain fog, chronic fatigue, low moods, sugar cravings, obesity, skin conditions, type 2 diabetes, polycystic ovary syndrome (PCOS), and non-alcoholic fatty liver disease.

Th food you choose impacts your glucose levels the most. Eating sweets and refined carbs alone on an empty stomach would cause the highest glucose spikes and drops, feeling tired shortly afterward. However, adding fibre, protein, or healthy fats can help stabilise your glucose levels and provide steady energy for longer periods of time.. Moreover, regular physical activity also helps to regulate glucose levels. Muscles need glucose to work, so having a simple walk or 10 minutes of moderate exercise after a meal would stabilise the curve.

These are the main principles to prevent or reverse conditions related to unhealthy blood sugar levels, but many more factors and techniques can also affect. Here you is a list of tips to help you with this.

- Don't consume sweets or refined carbs alone; pair them with fibre, protein or healthy fats.

- Walk or do moderate exercise for 10 minutes after a meal.

- Incorporate vinegar into your salads, consume a tbsp of apple cider vinegar before a meal, or add cinnamon to yogurt, desserts, or tea.

- The order you eat foods in a meal matters—start with vegetables (fibre) and save sweets for dessert.

- Manage stress and prioritise your sleep, as imbalances in both can affect glucose levels, causing irregular spikes.

- Women are more sensitive to blood sugar levels fluctuations and sweet cravings during their period and the previous two weeks. Be mindful of these principles, maintain a regular eating schedule, and get more rest during that phase.

- A breakfast rich in protein helps to regulate blood sugar levels throughout your day, while sweet options have the opposite effect.

3.8. Mind your gut health

Gut health is essential for our physical and mental well-being, as discussed in previous sections. Many modern health issues such as chronic fatigue, IBS, autoimmune conditions, and behavioural problems may have their origins in the gut.

Taking care of your gut health involves minimising the factors that can harm it, while prioritising foods and habits that can repair the gut lining and restore its balance. It requires a multi-factor approach to improve your lifestyle, which may include an initial phase focusing on healing for specific issues, followed by a maintenance phase.

Start with quality sleep from 7 - 9 hours to help your body heal and repair itself. Manage stress and include resting as some of your priorities. And do regular physical activity as well.

When it comes to food choices, boost your fibre intake with a variety of vegetables and colours, as well as flaxseeds, chia seeds, psyllium husks, and legumes. Include fermenting food sources of good bacteria or probiotics, such as kefir, yogurt, kombucha, kimchi, pickles, miso, Natto, tempeh, and sauerkraut. Add healthy fats regularly, such as Omega-3 fish and walnuts. And include foods with gut-healing properties like aloe vera, bone broth, collagen, pollen, and honey.

Reduce ultra-processed and junk foods, refined sugar, refined vegetable oils, alcohol, medicaments (e.g., antibiotics, acid blockers, or hormonal birth control.), smoking, and exposure to toxins. Consume gluten and conventional dairy in moderation as excessive intake may lead to gut imbalances. And if you experience any symptoms, consider an elimination diet to find out which foods and factors may be causing them, and explore alternatives options that work well for your body.

3.9. Supporting brain and nervous system

We know our bodies are complex designs and that food is a major factor that changes our chemistry. Food affects our moods, emotions, and brain performance. Our ability to solve problems, see the bigger picture, cope with emotions, rearrange concepts, create new ones, or feel inspired, is connected to our brain health and nervous system. We can work together in harmony with our bodies as an excellent team to support its needs at all levels, instead of putting it out of balance. Good nutrition and sleep become even more important in moments of emotional stress, work deadlines, exams, or intense mental activity. Paradoxically, is it when we often overlook them the most. In practice, we may not do them all perfectly, but we should try not to neglect any area completely, and it will surely pay off..

Less of what puts the body out of balance or harms it:

- Refined sugar and products with hidden added sugar
- Ultra-processed and junk foods
- Alcohol and smoking
- Sleep deprivation

More of the conditions and nutrients that support it:

- Quality sleep, rest, and fun time
- Vegetables and whole foods
- Mushrooms, avocados, eggs, berries, bananas
- Lentils, beans, chickpeas, quinoa, whole grains, nuts, and seeds
- Brain boosters: ginger, ginseng, turmeric, and cocoa
- Omega 3 fats: sardines, tuna, salmon, flaxseeds, and walnuts
- Probiotics: kimchi, kefir, yogurt, tempeh, miso, and pickles
- Physical activity, fun, and meaningful connections

Fats: The brain is primarily made of fat, and it needs it to thrive. Modern diets often have unbalanced ratios of different types, with too much saturated and Omega 6 fats, and a deficiency of Omega 3. Omega 3 is essential for brain and nervous system development, preserving mental health, and supporting the immune system. Good sources of healthy fat are nuts, seeds, avocados, olive oil, egg yolks, salmon, sardines, tuna, and mackerel.

Micronutrients: Nutrient deficiencies are very common nowadays due to the low nutritional value of ultra-processed foods. Vitamins and minerals are essential for all body functions, including those of the brain, nervous system, and energy production. For example, iron and B vitamins deficiencies can impact your vitality and mood. Nutrient-dense food sources are whole foods like vegetables, mushrooms, nuts, whole grains, fish, meat, and avocados.

Gut health: The gut and the brain are directly connected through the gut-brain axis, and the balance of those bacteria is important for mental and physical performance. Taking care of gut health involves reducing medicaments, stress, and alcohol, while including veggies, fibre, probiotics, fermented foods, and sleep.

Sleep: Sleep is an essential repair and recovery process of both the body and mind. The culture of neglecting it for more productivity is counteractive, as it makes us less efficient, more tired, less creative, and more susceptible to illness.

Movement: Humans are designed to move regularly for both physical and mental health. Physical activity has been proven to be a very effective remedy for preventing and treating depression and emotional problems.

3.10 How to understand food labels

Most health claims on the front of a package are misleading and just a part of marketing. Therefore, to make informed choices, it is important to look at the back and read the nutritional labels. These labels provide lots of information and have evolved to become more meaningful. Here are some guidelines to help you better understand food labels and choose the healthiest brands for your needs.

Ingredients list

Order: Ingredients are listed in the order of their predominance in the product. The first three or four are usually in the highest amounts, followed in descending order by the rest.

Names: Sugars, artificial ingredients, and trans fats may appear on food labels under different names. You can find the most common ones in the tables below. Remember, the fewer, the better.

Added sugars	Corn syrup, high-fructose corn syrup, fruit juice, maltose, dextrose, sucrose, honey, maple, or any syrup.
Trans fats	Partially hydrogenated oil, or hydrogenated vegetable oil (e.g. partially hydrogenated cottonseed oil).
Artificial ingredients	Artificial flavours, food additives, artificial sweeteners, E-xxx (e.g. E100), sodium benzoate, sodium nitrite, and monosodium glutamate.

- E-XXX are codes for substances permitted in the food industry. For example, E100-E199 are color codes, E200-E299 are preservatives codes, E300-E399 are antioxidants codes, etc. They are not all necessarily bad for health but don't provide nutritional value. However, as a general rule, fewer is better.

- Trans fats should be avoided. Margarine has high concentrations, and it can also be found in some industrial pastries, cakes, microwave popcorn, and deep-fried foods. Denmark was the first country to ban them in 2003.

- Products containing gluten, nuts, or other foods that trigger allergies will state this at the end of their ingredient list. Some foods are naturally gluten-free, such as, oats, but if they are produced in the same place as wheat or barley, they can become contaminated and contain gluten.

Here are two examples of cookies and their ingredients. Notice how the difference between brands of similar foods can be significant. The first one contains trans fats, added sugars, and artificial ingredients, while the last one doesn't, making it a better choice.

Examples

Cookies 1: wheat flour, water, soybean oil, sugar, partially hydrogenated cottonseed oil, salt, baking soda, high fructose corn syrup, soy lecithin, malted barley flour, natural flavour. Contains wheat and soy.

Cookies 2: wheat flour, chocolate chips, cane sugar, butter (milk), eggs, potato starch, vanilla, salt, xanthan gum, baking soda. Contains gluten and milk ingredients.

- The serving size is the amount of food the nutrient information is based on. When comparing brands, ensure that they are based on the same serving size.

- The % Daily Value is the percentage of the recommended daily value of a specific nutrient that a serving of food provides.

- A food is considered a good source of a particular nutrient when it provides at least 10 to 19% of the Daily Value per serving.

- Foods with low-calorie content contain 40 calories or less per serving size.

- Some countries use colour-coded labels to make them more intuitive and easy to understand. These usually indicate the quantity of sodium, saturated fat, and sugars.

- The "5–20" rule is a general guide to eating foods in the proper proportions. Instead of defining food as good or bad, the rule recommends choosing foods low in saturated fats, cholesterol, and sodium (less than 5% DV). Low and high DV is defined as:

    Low Daily Value (DV): less than 5%
    High Daily Value (DV): more than 20%

- Reduce high sugar foods, and consider that the difference between brands for the same food can be substantial especially for yogurts, juices, sauces, cereal packages, energy drinks, and plant-based products. You can visualise how much sugar a food contains, knowing that 4g of sugar equals one teaspoon.

    High sugar content: more than 22.5 g per 100 g
    Low sugar content: less than 5 g per 100 gr

‣ Protein is usually given in grams per serving size. The general recommendation is to include a serving of protein in each meal, which depends on each person, but it is usually from 20 g to 30 g.

‣ The recommendation for fat intake is to reduce consumption of foods high in saturated fat and increase intake of unsaturated fats. Reduce Omega 6 and increase Omega 3 intake, particularly for inflammatory conditions.

‣ Total carbohydrates on food labels are indicated in grams per serving size, and this value includes sugars, starches, and fibre. The general recommendation is to choose more complex carbs (such as whole grains and legumes instead of refined grains), increase fibre intake (for example, through vegetables), and reduce processed sugars (for instance, sweetened drinks).

‣ Choose products that have more variety and higher content of minerals and vitamins. These nutrients are needed in small quantities, and their amounts are indicated as the %DV (daily recommended value) on food labels. Note that if the content is < 5% DV, it is a very low source of that nutrient and may not be relevant.

‣ Fortified foods are products that have additional minerals and vitamins added to them. The most common nutrients added to these products are B12, calcium, and vitamin D. If you follow a plant-based diet, these products can be a good addition. Some other common fortified foods include vegetable milks, orange juice, dairy, and plant-based products.

Women are not supposed to have the same strengths or feel the same way every day of the month. They are cyclical beings. The hormonal fluctuations during each phase of the cycle affect everything else, including the body's blood sugar levels, physical strength, moods, concentration, sleep, cravings, and sociability. Living in harmony and sync with the body's needs would make everything easier, adapting her rhythm and schedule to her nature.

Keeping track of emotions and changes for a few months is a great way to discover how they affect her and possible patterns that previously passed unnoticed or caused unnecessary conflict in the past. She may realise that by the end of her cycle, she experiences more cravings, needs extra rest or quiet time, or doesn't feel like socialising.

In terms of nutrition and exercise, the hormonal and physical changes by the end of the cycle make her body require more calories and nutritional needs, become more sensitive to long periods of fasting, and experience higher fluctuations in blood sugar levels. It's important to consume more fibre, extra veggies, healthy fats, protein, and nutritionally dense foods, while limiting intake of junk food. Setting social boundaries, slowing down, finding moments of stillness, and prioritising rest can help support both the body and mind.

However, the first half of the cycle is probably a more active and naturally outgoing period. There is a healthy balance between play and rest, introspection and extroversion, and creative and productivity. Ignoring the body's needs or setting goals against your nature can make life more difficult or exhausting. If it feels too challenging, consider slowing down and giving yourself time and space. Clarity of vision and peace usually emerge during moments of stillness.

3.12. Daily practical tips

Accessibility to nutritious food and simplifying the practical application is essential for creating lasting changes, forming new habits, and integrating new normals as part of your life.

- Shop for vegetables and prepare them in advance. Wash, chop, and pre-cook them if necessary. Store them in containers so they're ready to use in your cooking or as a healthy snack.

- Replace processed sauces with more spices and herbs, such as black pepper, chili, curry, rosemary, parsley, coriander, basil, thyme, mint, oregano, cumin, turmeric, paprika, and ginger. They also have beneficial properties!

- Drink plain water instead of processed or sugary drinks.

- Have savoury breakfasts with protein and fibre for more stable energy and to stay satiated throughout your day.

- Check the labels on processed products and ingredients list on menus to choose healthier brands and restaurants. Differences between brands can be relevant in dairy, cereals, coffee mixes, chocolates, sauces, spreads, and ready-to-eat meals.

- Make healthy food accessible and visible, and keep the junk options out of sight. This will help you create new habits if temptations or triggers are not nearby, at least for a while.

- Make mental well-being and personal growth a priority, as imbalances can lead to health problems. When the mind, body, and spirit are aligned, most diseases cannot occur.

4. Modern Food Trends

Food is trendy today, which makes more people to rethink their habits and what they consume. While this is positive, the number of products and information may also be overwhelming. Self-education has become even more important with so many choices and contradictory messages. It's essential to be able to understand and interpret information without feeling it too complicated and be discouraged.

When the goal is to improve health and well-being, the main trends include consuming fewer highly processed products, less refined carbs and added sugars, and more nutrient-dense foods and veggies. Following this, the food pyramid is also evolving in this direction.

However, the most important factor is not just the dietary approach, but rather how to consistently implement these changes and shift habits behaviours. Perfection isn' necessary, but maintaining consistency in the long run is crucial.

All weight loss diets are based on the principle of creating a negative energy balance, which means eating fewer calories than physically needed. However, this equation is complex and depends on various factors, such as hormonal changes and age, and not all calories are the same. Therefore, the healthier method is to focus on consuming most of your calories from unprocessed nutrient-dense foods and tailor them to your conditions, which will make you feel better overall.

In real life, it is a multi-dimensional journey to understand how your choices and lifestyle affect you, the factors that limit you, and evolve. This is an ongoing holistic approach, as you will likely need to change habits and ideas, and continuously adapt them in the long term.

4.2. Vegan, vegetarian, and flexitarian

Vegan diets exclude all foods of animal origin. Vegetarian diets exclude foods of animal origin, with the exception of eggs, honey, and dairy. And, flexitarian diets primarily consist of vegetables and plant-based foods but also include meat and animal products in moderation.

The main guideline is to include more unprocessed and nutrient-dense foods while reducing junk, regardless of your dietary approach. Also, prioritise your sleep, physical activity, and mental well-being, and you will definitely feel better.

Here are some considerations and vegetarian alternatives to prevent possible nutrient deficiencies in the long term.

Calcium   Vitamin D   Magnesium   Iron

▸ Calcium, magnesium, and vitamin D are essential nutrients for building up and maintaining bone health, besides being part of more than 300 other functions for your well-being.

▸ Calcium: dairy, firm tofu, soybeans, beans, broccoli, green leafy vegetables, tempeh, almonds, and fortified foods (e.g., plant-based milk and orange juice).

▸ Vitamin D: egg yolks and fortified foods. The body can synthesize it from sunlight. Therefore countries with a lack of sunlight and vegan diets may need supplementation.

▸ Magnesium: whole grains, edamame, spinach, dark chocolate, almonds, cashews, peanuts, quinoa, avocado, and black beans.

Protein is composed of amino acids, some of which the body can't make and must obtain from food—these are known as essential amino acids. Animal protein is considered complete because it contains all of these, unlike most plant-based sources. However, by combining different plant-based foods, it is possible to create a complete protein source, as you can see below.

In addition to protein, iron and B12 are also nutrients mostly from animal origin, but here you can find plant-based alternatives.

- Iron: beans, chickpeas, lentils, potatoes, soybeans, pumpkin seeds, cashews, chia, quinoa, spinach, kale, figs, dried apricots, raisins, tofu, and fortified foods.

- B12: egg yolks, dairy, and fortified foods with B12 (e.g., cereals and milk). However, vegan diets need B12 supplementation.

- Complete protein sources: all dairy (e.g., milk, yogurt, curd, kefir, and cheese). Egg whites for vegetarian diets. And strictly plant-based options are tofu, seitan, tempeh, edamame, soybeans, soy milk, hemp seeds, chia seeds, green peas, quinoa, buckwheat, hemp seeds, and amaranth.

- Complete protein combinations: grains with legumes (e.g., rice and lentils, rice and beans, tahini on bread, hummus on pita, or peanut butter toast). And, legumes or grains with nuts and seeds (e.g., oatmeal with almonds and walnuts, a multi-seed bread toast with almond butter, or peanuts and seeds).

4.3. Sugar and glycemic index

The effects of excessive refined sugar are already well-known today. It provides low-quality or "empty calories" with little nutritional value, which can lead to nutritional deficiencies, obesity, brain fog, mood swings, and long-term health issues, such as type 2 diabetes, cardiovascular problems, and PCOS.

Refined or white sugar is often added to processed products to enhance the flavour at a low cost, resulting in hyper-palatable foods that are easy to overeat and have addictive properties, such as fast food, sweetened drinks, or most chocolate bars. However, there is a rising awareness of this issue, and "sugar-free" has become a new trend. Nowadays, more and more people check nutritional labels, have access to more education, and there are more alternatives in the market, like "conscious" brands.

However, not all sugars are the same. There are also fewer processed sugars like coconut sugar and jaggery, and natural ones also contain fibre, vitamins, and health properties, such fruits and honey. The recommendation is to consume the less processed sugar, while applying moderation with the natural ones.

In practice, the effect that sugar has on the body depends on the other nutrients it is consumed with. For example, fibre and protein make blood sugar levels rise slower while providing a more steady release of energy, preventing a "sugar crash" later on. Eating a sweet dessert after a balanced meal does not have the same effect as snacking on sweets between meals. The way you combine foods matters too.

The glycemic index, or GI, is a parameter created to measure this, and it describes how fast sugar is released into the blood.

GI values are measured on a scale from 0 to 100, with white sugar being assigned a GI of 100. In practice, low GI lead to more stable energy, while those with higher GI values can result in unhealthier blood sugar fluctuations and energy levels throughout the day.

However, note that the total GI of a meal depends on the combination of foods. Including fibre, protein, and good fats lower the total GI, making the GI of each individual food less significant. Considering this, you can use the following list as a guide to consume high-GI foods in moderation and pair them with lower-GI options, especially those high in fibre.

Glycemic Index (GI)

Low GI: less than 55

All leafy and non-starchy vegetables, nuts, seeds, flaxseeds and psyllium husks (fibre sources), beans, lentils, chickpeas, quinoa, yams, buckwheat, brown rice, dairy, soy milk, soybeans, eggs, oatmeal crackers, apples, berries, oranges, pears, and peaches.

Medium GI: between 55 and 69

Beetroot, taro, wholemeal rye, porridge, couscous, basmati rice, chapati, roti, corn tortilla, barley, spaghetti, rice noodles, porridge, muesli, seeded or brown bread, bananas, plantain, raisins, papaya, pineapple, figs.

High GI: more than 69

White wheat bread, most cakes and pastries, ice cream, rice crackers, pumpkin, parsnips, most breakfast cereals, white and glutinous rice, rice milk, tapioca, mashed potatoes, watermelon, very ripe tropical fruits, and dried fruits.

4.4. How to deal with sweet cravings

After discussing some benefits of reducing sugars, it's time to talk about the practice. Changing our habits and diet can present both practical and emotional challenges in real life. These are the main factors that will determine what changes you will actually implement.

Alternatives to white sugar: Dried fruits, beetroot, pumpkin, honey, jaggery, raw cane sugar, coconut sugar, agave nectar, maple syrup. Sugar-free alternatives: Stevia, xylitol,

A good start is first replacing sweets with healthier options. Here you have two lists of alternatives to replace white sugar in your cooking or go for healthy snacks to satisfy food cravings.

1 tsp honey, walnuts, and cinnamon
1 date and a walnut
A handful of nuts and seeds
Fresh fruit or a smoothie with nuts
Boiled eggs with salt and pepper
1-2 tsp nut butter on wholegrain toast
Avocado or guacamole with veggies
Pita with hummus or tahini
Unsweetened yogurt with flaxseeds

The other aspect of dealing with cravings is observing their triggers and reasons. You may need to balance your main meals so you are not hungry soon afterward or to prevent a "sugar crash." Practice other ways to cope with challenging emotions. Reduce stress in your life and do activities to relieve it. Or transform your relationship with food. Mindful eating can help to observe these aspects, create new habits. And remember that new habits always take time, so be patient.

Food intolerances and allergies have risen in recent years, especially gluten and lactose intolerances. Besides being a trend that people may follow in the hope of health benefits, the diagnosed cases have also increased, and they are often developed later in life during adulthood.

We are continually discovering new aspects about the physical effect of certain foods under different conditions. Additionally, factors such as increased pesticide and medicine use, higher levels of contamination and stress, and a higher incidence of gut health problems are likely to have contributed to this modern phenomenon.

The symptoms usually include bloating, tiredness or chronic fatigue, headaches, brain fog, skin conditions, inflammatory flares, weight loss, and low vitality. However, these are also symptoms of many other conditions. In practice, elimination diets are often the best approach to determine if you would feel better without these products.

If you feel unwell, it's very important to investigate for the underlying causes and consider food intolerances as one of the potential factors. Don't dismiss feeling tired, in pain, or uninspired as normal—while it may be common, it is not normal. Your body wants you to thrive, and will do it the more you live in harmony with its natural rhythm and needs, not against them.

The health of your digestive system and gut should become a priority if you experience food intolerance symptoms. Your body needs specific conditions to properly digest and absorb nutrients, such as adequate enzymes, a balanced gut flora, certain levels of digestive juices, and a healthy gut linen. When any of these factor are persistently out of balance, symptoms may occur.

In this section, you can find an overview of the most common intolerances nowadays, which are dairy (lactose or casein) and gluten.

Lactose

Lactose is the sugar found in animal milk, which the body can digest thanks to a specific enzyme. The amount of these enzymes decreases during adulthood, making it less easy for the body to process and maybe causing lactose intolerant. An alternative is to consume plant-based milk made from nuts and grains, which are naturally lactose-free. However, check the ingredients of these products as they often contain added sugars or additives to enhance the flavour.

Casein

Casein is a type of protein in milk that can cause inflammatory reactions if the body has difficulty breaking it down. It is more common in children, especially if they are not breastfed, but it often disappears through in adulthood.

Gluten

Gluten is a type of protein present in some cereals like wheat, rye, and barley, and therefore in most bread, pasta, and pastries. Gluten intolerance is called celiac disease. However, many other conditions are considered within the spectrum of gluten sensitivity and would also benefit from reducing its intake. Some cases are irritable bowel syndrome (IBS), autism, depression, and autoimmune conditions.

For reference, gluten sources include wheat, rye, barley, and malt, while gluten-free sources are rice, cassava, corn, soy, potatoes, tapioca, beans, quinoa, millet, amaranth, yucca, all nuts and seeds, nut flours, and gluten-free oats.

4.6. Intermittent Fasting

The potential benefits and properties of fasting have made it more popular in recent years. Some studies suggest that it may help lose weight, regulate insulin levels and blood pressure, reduce triglycerides and inflammation, promote cell regeneration, and slow down the aging process. Intermittent fasting (IF) is the most common approach, involving a daily fasting window of 12 - 16 hours, often consisting of having early dinners or skipping breakfast.

During fasting, the body starts to use its fat reserves, making IF a popular choice for those looking to lose body fat. However, it's important to consider potential side effects and other factors to estimate if it's the right option for you. First, focusing on quality nutrition and eating more unprocessed, nutrient-dense foods is the primary step in any nutritional approach, regardless of meal timing. Second, balancing the total energy intake and the energy expenditure (for example, through increased physical activity) is crucial in determining weight fluctuations. And lastly, drastic changes in meal schedule or feeling restricted can impact your social or family life, mental well-being, and the relationship with food, all of which are very important for long-term health.

Besides this, women are more sensitive to fasting at different phases of their monthly cycle due to the unique hormonal changes. However, most research has focused on men or menopausal women. Moreover, the benefits of cell regeneration come with longer fasts, but this may lead to side effects like nutrient deficiencies or impact bone health.

In the end, the effects of fasting can vary a lot from person to person and depend on individual health conditions, the balance of benefits versus side effects, and how it is implemented in practice.

4.7. Keto and low-carb diets

Ketogenic is a metabolic state in which your body uses fat for fuel instead of carbs. This state can be reached by limiting the daily carbs intake to 20-50 grams, which usually accounts for about 10% of the daily calorie intake. The remaining calories come from protein and healthy fats, such as eggs, meat, fish, nuts, and unrefined oils. Also, intermittent fasting can help the body enter ketosis more quickly.

Low-carb diets allow for a higher carb intake, up to 30% of the total daily calories, making them less restrictive and more suitable for the long term. These diets also focus on reducing bread, pastries, pasta, sweets, and refined carbs while including plenty of protein and fats. However, they generally include more vegetables and fruits, which makes them higher in fibre and micronutrients.

Both approaches claim to help with losing body fat, regulating blood sugar levels, treating type 2 diabetes or other insulin-related conditions like PCOS, and feeling more energetic and focused. However, side effects can vary depending on each person, including fatigue, headache, sleep problems, hormonal imbalances, poor concentration, or the development of food aversions.

Therefore, the right dietary approach must be decided according to the condition to treat or goal to pursue, life circumstances, and individual physical needs. For example, women tend to require a higher intake of healthy carbs to maintain general well-being, while some people who need to lose weight may thrive with a keto diet.

As a general recommendation, extreme or restrictive approaches are often suitable only for a short period, while balance and moderation are the healthiest directions for the long term.

4.8. What are super foods?

Foods that are very nutrient-dense are known as superfoods, which means that they are a source of lots of the goodness your body needs. They are not newly discovered, they have been used since the ancient times, and even some were daily foods in those days.

Superfoods are very rich in different nutrients, like minerals, vitamins, antioxidants, proteins, fibre, and carbs, and fibre, and offer various health benefits. Nowadays, with the rise of monoculture farming and pesticide use, there is a concern that regular foods may be losing their nutritional value, leading to the increased popularity and prices of superfoods.

We can consider most natural, unprocessed foods as superfoods, such as eggs, raw nuts, scallops, salmon, sardines, spinach, cauliflower, pumpkin, mushrooms, beans, lentils, chickpeas, ginger, berries, kefir, and yogurt. You don't need to spend lots of money to be healthy or do complicated things. Choosing a balanced diet based mainly on whole foods is the main step. You can sometimes complement this with some of the trendy superfoods as boosters, but not to make up for excesses, deficiencies, or lack of consistency with good habits.

In the following pages, you can find an overview of some popular superfoods along with a brief overview history. These are some of the oldest foods consumed worldwide, and each country has its local products considered superfoods. As a general guideline, "the more local you consume, the better." Additionally, if you have access to seasonal products, they are even more nutritious, fresher, and healthier.

- Wheatgrass, chlorella, spirulina, and seaweed are excellent sources of chlorophyll, antioxidants, vitamins, and minerals. They have many properties, including detoxifying your system, boosting the immune system, preventing cancer, and rejuvenating the skin. They come from all over the world. More concretely, spirulina is known to have been consumed by the Aztecs in Mexico, chlorella and seaweed have their roots in Japan, and wheatgrass is the oldest, having been used by the Egyptians in Mesopotamia.

- Avocados are a source of healthy fats and various vitamins, such as vitamins C, E, and D. They are recommended for support ing brain health and mental well-being, the cardiovascular system, and hormonal balance, and preserving bones and muscles. Avocados originated in Mexico around 10,000 years ago, and the Aztecs invented guacamole. Nowadays, you can still eat it fresh in every market and restaurant in Mexico.

- Maca is a root that provides carbohydrates and energy to boost physical performance and strength. It is also considered to have properties to support higher moods, immunity, and fertility. Maca comes from Peru and Bolivia, where Inca soldiers were said to have carried it into battles to gain power and endurance.

- Green tea is considered one of the healthiest drink in the world due to its high antioxidant content. It is a staple in traditional Chinese medicine and is considered to have properties to reduce inflammatory conditions, slow down aging, support brain health, help body fat loss, and prevent cancer. Green tea originated in China almost 5,000 years ago and remains popular worldwide today.

▸ Broccoli is one of the superfoods in the vegetable kingdom. It is a source of vitamin K, C, folic acid, potassium, fibre, calcium, and phytonutrients. It is known for its many health properties, such as being an antioxidant and anti-inflammatory, supporting liver cleansing, protecting the heart, and helping rejuvenate the skin. Broccoli is native to the Mediterranean and was a valuable food during the Roman Empire. The Italians introduced it to the US only later in the 20th century.

▸ Chia seeds come from Central and South America, and legends say that Aztecs and Mayans used them as a source of energy. They contain complete protein, making them an excellent choice for plant-based diets, and are also a good source of fibre and Omega-3 fats. As previously explained, Omega-3 is recommended to support the brain, the immune system, gut health, and the treatment of inflammatory conditions.

▸ Flax seeds are an excellent source of fibre and Omega-3 fats. They are best to consume ground, but can also be soaked overnight. Adding just 1-2 tbsps a day in yogurt, milk, smoothies, or even soup is a great healthy habit for gut health and overall well-being. The origin of flax seeds is unclear, but some believe they are native to Egypt.

▸ Quinoa, originally from South America, was a staple food back in those days and has made a comeback in recent years with the rise of plant-based diets. It is a gluten-free source of complete protein, making it ideal for vegans, vegetarians, and people with gluten intolerances. It is also rich in fibre, B vitamins, magnesium, and healthy complex carbs.

- Berries and goji berries are very rich in antioxidants and vitamin C, which support the immune system and fight free radicals. Although they sound similar, they come from different places: blueberries are from North America, while goji berries are from China.

- Acai berries are very high in antioxidants and health-promoting properties, containing lots of fibre, B vitamins, magnesium, potassium, and phosphorus. Studies show that they may help improve cognitive function and blood sugar levels, boost the immune system, and slow down aging. Originally from Central and South America, especially Brazil, acai berries are now available worldwide in powder form, ready to mix into smoothies or for the famous "acai bowl."

- Cacao contains antioxidants, magnesium, calcium, and iron, which can help with muscle recovery, relaxation, cardiovascular health, sleep, energy levels, and supporting bone health. Cacao is also known for naturally elevating moods and is recommended for happier lives. It comes from Central and South America and has been consumed for over 4,000 years by cultures in the Yucatán, like the Mayans.

- Bone broth is one of the best sources of gelatin and collagen protein, which are beneficial for connective tissues and gut health. It contains calcium, magnesium, phosphorus, silicon, sulfur, and other compounds like chondroitin sulfate and glucosamine that benefit joints, the digestive system, and skin. Bone broth has been used in traditional Chinese medicine for over 2500 years and has become part of most Asian cuisines.

You are your genes, but not entirely. Some of your characteristics are there, like lines in the code of information inside the world of DNA. They also give the instructions for making the building blocks that build your body, so literally, they define your structure. However, much about the world of DNA remains a mystery yet to be discovered.

The DNA encodes millions of possibilities, of which only a few are expressed, and many factors can impact this—including what you eat. Does it mean that your genes can change? In a way, yes! The field of research on how food and environmental conditions interact with gene expression is called nutrigenomics.

Imagine having genes that can be activated based on various factors, such as lifestyle and diet. It's like a program with instructions that can engage one gene or another depending on the input, with millions of possibilities and conditions that can determine which gene is expressed.

For example, broccoli contains compounds that can activate a specific gene in the liver that detoxifies toxins, while cooked tomatoes could deactivate genes that reduce the risk of prostate cancer. Therefore, this is why we are not just your genes after all. Our genetic makeup is more complex than a fixed equation we inherit at birth.

The important lesson here is that you have more possibilities at hand than you might have realised to improve your well-being, regardless of your genetic makeup. Our DNA, which we once believed to be a fixed, predetermined equation, may actually be fluid and capable of transformation over time based on our lifestyle. Isn't that amazing?

5. Food as Medicine

5.1. Natural treatments for parasites

Papaya seeds

Papaya seeds are considered to have properties that can help treat parasites and fight dengue. They can be consumed fresh or dried, and a couple of spoonfuls a day is enough. Consuming too many seeds may cause nausea or other side effects. If treating parasites, take the papaya seeds with a low-sugar diet, and increase your intake of vegetables, lemon, and water.

Pumpkin seeds

Pumpkin seeds contain a substance called cucurbitacin, which has properties that may help treat worms and other parasites by paralysing them so they can be expelled from the body. They need to be eaten raw, not fried or roasted. Besides that, they are source of healthy fats and iron.

Oregano oil

Oregano oil is considered to have also anti-parasitic properties. Mix 2 or 3 drops of it in water with freshly squeezed lemon, and drink it about three times a day.

Garlic

Garlic is popular for its beneficial and healing properties, including as part of parasite treatment. It needs to be eaten raw, which can be challenging at first. You can start with one crushed clove in a juice and increase the dose as you slowly get used to it.

Aloe vera

Aloe vera has properties that can help heal wounds, including ulcers, and it is used as part of the treatment for acid reflux. It is also recommended for healing the gut lining in conditions such as the leaky gut, prevent constipation, and for its high levels of antioxidants. You can add the pulp from aloe vera in smoothies, or find the juice in health shops and drink it with water in the morning. Additionally, a freshly sliced stalk can be applied to the skin for wounds or used as a shampoo for a dry scalp.

Papaya

Papaya also has soothing properties that can help to heal wounds. It is used as part of the treatment for ulcers, acid reflux, and gut health conditions. It is an excellent option for everyone for its rich content of vitamins and antioxidants, especially when dealing with digestive problems or constipation.

Yogurt

Yogurt has calming properties for the stomach, is easy to digest, and can help to restore gut bacteria. It has traditionally the choice for delicate stomachs or during sickness.

Bananas and oatmeal

Bananas and oatmeal have soothing properties for the digestive tract to relieve acid reflux and support gut health. They are recommended for vomiting or diarrhea, especially bananas to help rehydrate. Also, it is also best to reduce the following foods: deep-fried, alcohol, chocolate, caffeine, added sugars, and fatty foods.

5.3. Sleeping difficulties

The quality and quantity of your sleep affect your overall well-being, both physically and mentally. While you sleep, your body repairs itself, and your mind processes the events of the day. Therefore, if you have difficulties with sleep, it's important to take care of them and not leave them untreated. The emphasis on efficiency and productivity in today's fast-paced world has led to a decrease in the amount of sleep people get, which has taken a toll on our health.

The recommended sleep duration is from 7 to 9 hours, with about 1-2 hours of deep sleep. This can vary based on factors such as age and stress. Every night, you have several consecutive cycles of NREM (non-rapid eye movement) and REM (rapid eye movement) sleep.

NREM is the deep sleep phase when the body optimises its physical balance, strengthens the immune system, regenerates cells, and boosts memory skills. Then, during the REM or dreaming phase, information and experiences are processed and integrated, associations are built, insights happen, and creativity is enhanced. Hence, if you need to make big decisions, wait first for a good night of sleep to see the bigger picture.

Several lifestyle and dietary factors regulate your sleep cycles and the hormones that determine when you fall asleep. Some of them include having enough sunlight exposure, regular physical activity, stress management, eating mainly unprocessed and nutrient-dense foods, and avoiding nutrient deficiencies.

Regarding dietary approaches, lighter early dinners with less refined carbs and sugars can help your body to rest. Staying too hungry at night during your fasting window may keep you awake, and too much alcohol has a sedative effect that disrupts your sleep cycles, reducing the REM phase. In addition, the following foods are considered to support relaxation and optimise sleep quality: almonds, walnuts, Omega-3 fish, cottage cheese, turkey, kiwis, hot milk with cinnamon, chamomile, and valerian tea with honey. Below, you will find a list of natural practices and tips to help you sleep better.

- Direct exposure to morning sunlight without sunglasses
- Doing regular physical activity
- Changing blue lights with warm lights
- Having the last coffee at midday
- Skipping evening alcohol
- Using magnesium spray
- Including more Omega-3 foods
- Getting a feet bath with Epsom salts
- Gentle stretching before bedtime
- Listening to relaxing music
- Meditating or breathing slowly
- Having a warm shower before bedtime to relaxes the muscles
- Turning off gadgets one h before bedtime
- Moving your working schedule earlier
- Having a break from social media
- Drinking a valerian tea before bedtime
- Going to bed 9 hours before your waking up time
- Writing down all you have in your mind or what you need to do the day after to feel quieter

5.4. Tips for inflammatory conditions

Turmeric

Turmeric is widely used for its anti-inflammatory properties in the traditional Indian medicine known as Ayurveda. It is recommended to consume turmeric with black pepper or a source of good fat for better absorption by the body. This recipe of golden milk can be a good start: boil coconut milk, turmeric, honey, and additional spices like cinnamon, anise, and cloves.

Ginger

Ginger is also commonly used in many traditional medicines for its anti-inflammatory properties and to help with digestion. It can be added fresh to your dishes or shakes, or consumed as tea.

Cinnamon

Cinnamon is used in both Ayurveda and traditional Chinese medicine for its anti-inflammatory properties and its ability to help regulate blood sugar levels. It can be added to desserts, yogurts, milk, porridge, or boiled in tea.

Pineapples, Grapefruit, and Berries

Fruits are rich in vitamins and antioxidants, and some may also have anti-inflammatory properties. Pineapple, grapefruit, and blueberries are particularly beneficial.

Cocoa

Cocoa is considered to have anti-inflammatory properties and is a good source of magnesium, iron, and antioxidants. However, sweet chocolate or compound is not the same; go for real cocoa.

Green tea

Green tea has an important place in traditional Chinese medicine due to its numerous health benefits, including properties as an antioxidant, anti-inflammatory, and for cancer prevention.

Omega-3

Omega-3 is a very important type of fat that research has shown to have anti-inflammatory properties and play essential roles in brain health and the nervous system. Most modern diets are deficient and unbalanced in the ratio between Omega-3 and Omega-6 fats, which has inflammatory effects. Some good food sources to include more often are oily fish (such as salmon, tuna, sardines, and mackerel), walnuts, flax seeds, and chia seeds.

Foods to reduce

The natural treatment for inflammatory conditions involves not only knowing what to eat and do more of but also what to reduce. The the most common foods with inflammatory properties are junk foods, refined sugar, refined vegetable oils, most industrial cakes and pastries, sweetened drinks, refined flour like white bread (with exceptions such as sourdough bread), and alcohol.

Lifestyle

Food is just one factor that can impact inflammatory conditions. However, your lifestyle and habits also play a significant role in your overall health and triggering inflammation. Sleep deprivation, lack of movement, and especially excessive stress are important areas to balance. Therefore, try to adopt habits for better sleep, practice techniques for relieving stress, deal with external stressors, and make changes in your life, rearrange priorities, and move more.

5.5. Morning rituals

The first things you do when you wake up are important and create the conditions for the rest of the day, both physically and mentally. Starting with a positive attitude instead of negativity, feeling grateful instead of complaining, listening to music instead of the news, or just smiling while you shower—all these can set you in the right direction.

The same applies to your physical state. If you start overloading your body with sugars and processed foods, you will experience spiky blood sugar levels that will be more difficult to balance later. This will make you tired, sluggish, or demotivated and most probably lead to cravings or unhealthy choices throughout the day, creating a cycle that becomes increasingly difficult to break.

In the morning, your body comes from a fasting state, and the first thing to put in it should be water to clean and wake up your system, preferable warm water with lemon. You can also add aloe vera juice for its cleansing and gut-healing properties.

Next, you can have breakfast within one hour after waking up and make it savoury, mainly whole, nutrient-dense foods rich in protein and fibre. This can help regulate blood sugar and energy levels throughout the day, increase mental and physical performance, feel satiated for longer, and reduce food cravings.

In addition, some people feel better by extending the fasting window and skipping breakfast. This can be a good option as long as the other meals are balanced and don't lead to overeating later. However, most people would benefit more from having savoury breakfasts and light early dinners in the evening, but it ultimately depends on balancing social commitments, work schedules, and individual preferences.

- Healthy bread with a topping of protein: Healthy bread, such as rye, sourdough, seeded whole grain, or Ezekiel bread, is rich in fibre and contains more nutrients,

- Smoothies: They provide fibre, minerals, vitamins, antioxidants, and water. Add some nuts for good fats and fibre.

- Eggs: A couple of eggs cooked in any style and accompanied with avocado, toast, or sauté spinach with mushrooms.

- Nuts: If you are in a hurry, grab a handful of nuts and seeds to eat on the go. You can take a fruit to add more vitamins.

- Oats: Porridge with oats, nuts and seeds, cinnamon, and unsweetened milk. You can top it up with berries and cacao.

- Dairy: Unsweetened yogurt or kefir are great options, topped with fruits and nuts for the morning. Cheese, cottage, quark, and feta are good high-protein choices to eat with toast, a few oatcakes, or honey and walnuts.

- A wrap or sandwich: Fill it with green leaf salad, vegetables, guacamole, beans, or hummus. Use a tortilla, healthy bread, lettuce leaves, seaweed sheet, or pita.

- Granola or muesli: Granola is made with baked oats, nuts, and sugar or another sweetener, while muesli has less sugar and is not baked. In both cases, choose the one with more nuts and less sugar, and have it with milk, kefir, or yogurt.

- Fruit salad: Mix fruits (e.g., apples and berries) with plain yogurt, low-sugar muesli or granola, nuts, and seeds.

5.6. Medicinal foods in world traditions

Food builds up your physical body and can create the conditions for you to thrive or the opposite. While there there are various factors that influence your overall well-being and how you feel, the food you consume also affect your brain health, nervous system, and body chemistry. Therefore, it is not surprising that traditional medicines have long considered food as a treatment and medicine. While they can't replace a healthy, balanced diet and overall lifestyle—nothing can do—but they can boost your system and help with health conditions. Here are examples of such foods and their uses, many of which have been covered in previous chapters.

Ginger and Turmeric

Ginger and turmeric have been mentioned a few times because they are some of the most accessible products and both have impressive health benefits. They are considered to have properties to boost the immune system, help digestive processes, and relieve inflammation.

Ginger is widely used in Asian and Arabic traditions. It is recommended for motion and morning sickness, indigestion, headaches, flu, diarrhea, arthritis, and pain during menstruation. However, it is advised not to take it if suffering from high blood pressure.

Turmeric has been used in India and Ayurveda for over 2,500 years and is recommended for arthritis, anemia, diabetes, gallstones, poor circulation, and Alzheimer's prevention.

Cinnamon

This healthy spice comes from the Far East and has been present in Chinese traditions for centuries. It was also imported by the ancient Greeks for use in their medical practices. Cinnamon is considered to have beneficial properties including antioxidant, anti-inflammatory, anti-diabetic, anti-microbial, anti-cholesterol, immunity-boosting, and heart-protecting effects. As a result, it is recommended for helping regulating blood sugar levels, immune system conditions, muscle soreness, painful menstruation, regulating blood pressure, and treating infections.

Walnuts

Nuts are excellent sources of healthy fats and are considered superfood. They are a leading food in traditional Chinese medicine, often prescribed for cognitive abilities, preventing memory loss, dealing with immune system conditions, balancing cholesterol, and regulating blood sugar levels. More concretely, walnuts are especially rich in Omega-3 fats, which mean they may have anti-inflammatory, nervous system protective, and brain-boosting properties.

Garlic

Garlic is believe to have antibacterial, anti-viral, anti-cardiovascular disease, anti-diabetic, and anti-cancer properties. It is thought to originate from Central or South Asia and is advised for heart disease prevention, controlling high blood pressure and diabetes, and treating colds, infections, and parasites. The most effective form is to eat it raw in the morning or as black fermented garlic, which is easier to digest and has a pleasant taste. When using it for cooking, add it at the end to prevent it from burning.

Onions

Onions are considered to have properties such as anti-clotting, anti-coagulant, anti-diabetic, and anti-parasite. They are widely grown and used worldwide and are recommended for respiratory problems such as colds, coughs, bronchitis, asthma, parasites and infections, as well as for relieving excess gas and diabetes.

Lemons

Lemons are famous for their health benefits and high vitamin C content. They can support the immune system support, fight bacterial infections, and aid in detoxification. They are used in medicinal foods globally and are easily added to your regular diet.

Mushrooms

Mushrooms have held an important place in the traditional medicines of China and Japan. They belong to a unique kingdom of their own and there are thousands of edible classes, some of which have medicinal properties. They are considered nutrient-dense with antiviral and anti-inflammatory properties that support brain health, mental performance, and longevity. They are also recommended for treating infections, candida, diabetes, and arteriosclerosis.

Goji berries

Goji berries are excellent sources of antioxidants, which can aid in collagen production, protect the eyes, support detoxification processes, and improve skin conditions. They have been widely used in traditional Chinese medicine and are now popular as a superfood.

6. Eco and Sustainable

6.1. Laws of nature and interdependence

We are subject to laws that we can neither change nor evade, but we can observe and follow them. These are the laws of nature and are inherent to our existence. Being more in tune and harmony with them allows us to thrive, enhances our sensitivity and perception, and expand our life experience. Ignoring these laws does not make them disappear, and living disconnected from them is like swimming against the current, eventually leading to physical and mental imbalances.

One of them is the law of interdependence. This is the symbiotic relationship we share with everything in and around us, from the smallest unit of life in the body that performs certain functions for us, to our link with the rest of life and the earth. Ignoring this creates imbalances, while embracing it leads to a more fulfilling, joyful, magical, and harmonious life, as disconnection results in confusion.

In this world of interdependencies, all our choices have an impact, and we have the power to make positive contributions. Taking care of ourselves as much as to our surroundings may be essential to experience actual health and balance, and it may be part of what we are more than a mere personal choice. This involves caring for our bodies, the people around us, and the rest of nature.

Terms such as "Eco," "bio," "green," and "sustainable," besides being commercial trends, also reflect a growing awareness and the necessity for it. And, although the meanings of such labels can sometimes be misleading, the overall flow toward this direction is what truly matters.

6.2. Organic, natural and eco

There are many reasons to consume organic food, with health being the main one. However, there is confusion regarding the value of these foods are for their price and their feasibility on a large scale. This debate can feel overwhelming, and there isn't just a single answer, so let's explore how to make these choices without breaking the bank.

Firstly, the main benefit is avoiding the chemicals and pesticides that can have adverse effects on health. However, not all pesticides are the same, and each country decides which ones are allowed. Moreover, in legal terms, the definitions of organic, natural, or ecological can vary in different parts of the world, adding complexity to the issue.

The second aspect is food quality. The body needs nutrients from food, and this depends on the quality of the soil in which it's grown, as well as other conditions such as weather and sunlight. Non-organic foods are believed to have a lower concentration of nutrients for the same product, but the extent of this difference is not entirely clear.

Some guidelines for choosing your products include to prioritising unprocessed foods over ultra-processed ones, opting for local foods that are naturally fresher and more environmentally friendly, and if you can afford some organic foods, starting with organic versions of the foods most affected by pesticides (see a list in the next section). Then, if you have ticked all these boxes and have spare a budget, you can extend your shopping list to include more organic foods.

In places where there is no control, terms like "green," "natural," or "eco" on a package can mean anything, but prices can rise quickly when these labels are present. To help you with this, you can find some guidelines for these terms on the following page.

- The "Organic" label for vegetables and fruits require must compliance with official specifications. This means the soil is free of chemicals and pesticides for a certain number of years, and non-GMO (genetically modified organisms) seeds are used. This does not mean that no synthetic pesticides are used at all, only those that are allowed, and the list of permitted pesticides can change.

- For animals, the "Organic" label means they were raised in conditions that accommodate their natural behaviours, fed organic food, and not given antibiotics or hormones. Organic eggs must also come from chickens raised in these conditions.

- The use of the word "organic" is regulated by the United States Department of Agriculture (USDA). It can't be used on packages without an official certification, which guarantees that the product complies with the official standards.

- On products made from several ingredients, the USDA organic seal indicates that between 70% and 95% of the ingredients are organic.

- The term "Natural" denotes minimal processing and no artificial ingredients.

- The "Eco" and "Green" labels indicate that the product and its manufacturing process do not harm the environment. These labels apply varios products including food, clothing, packaging, household items, vehicles, and houses. It's important to note that these names are less regulated and are sometimes used falsely for marketing reasons.

We understand that choosing organic products can offer better quality and support sustainable farming practices and the environment. However, it can be expensive and concerns about quality of they are worthy may hold us back.

It's important to note that being healthy does not need to be expensive; it's more about balancing overall habits and lifestyle with small different daily choices. In addition to that, being organic does not automatically make food healthier. For instance, you are probably better off eating some non-organic papaya and nuts than a whole packet of organic and gluten-free cookies. Ultimately, eating healthier is more about habits and knowledge than money.

Also, certain foods are more affected by pesticides than others, so opting for organic versions of those foods can make a bigger difference. Generally, fruits and vegetables with a hard peel are freer of chemicals, like bananas, pumpkins, dragon fruit, avocados, kiwis, onions, pineapples, grapefruit, mangos, and sweet potatoes.

Here you can see "the Dirty Dozen" from the Environmental Working Group—a list of the foods with the highest load of pesticides, and therefore, most worth buying organic.

The Dirty Dozen

Strawberries

Apples

Nectarines

Peaches

Celery

Grapes

Cherries

Spinach

Tomatoes

Sweet bell peppers

Cherry tomatoes

Cucumbers

6.4. Adapt your diet to the weather

Adapting your diet to the weather and seasons is a central principle of most traditional medicines, such as Ayurveda. These practices believe that there is an innate intelligence in the rhythm of nature, which provides adequate products at different times of the year.

The body has different needs depending on the weather and the environment, and the soil naturally produces different foods at different months and in each climate around the world. However, with the modern possibility of consuming anything from anywhere at any time, we have forgotten this principle.

Generally, it is recommended to consume more fat and heavier meals in the cold season, eat lighter salads and fruits in hotter and drier climates, and try to buy seasonal and local products, which are often even cheaper.

6.5. Age, body type, and lifestyle

The diet that is right for you is likely to be different from someone else's. Factors such as your level of physical activity, age, gender, body type, and any hidden food intolerances play a role in determining your specific nutritional needs. It's important to consider and adjust your diet accordingly.

This topic is complex and could fill an entire book, and this section is just a note to encourage you to question and explore your own needs. Don't apply generic advice without adapting it to yourself, and pay attention to what your body is telling you. If you're not feeling well, you may need to change your diet or certain habits. Don't take feeling unwell as normal, keep open to question things.

6.6. Shop for local and seasonal products

Eating local and seasonal food is healthier for you, the planet, and the rest of nature. These foods are probably fresher, have fewer chemicals, more nutrients, and are better suite for the body's needs based on the weather and the season. Therefore, they're most likely good for you.

Moreover, by shopping locally, you reduce the need for transportation and the pollution it creates, and you also contribute to your local economy. So, it is also healthier for the planet and everyone else.

The truth is that not all small farmers who use organic methods can afford to get officially certified, and they may only sell on a small scale directly or at farmers' markets. Those are usually friendly social events, sometimes with music, secondhand items, or pop-up stalls, creating a fun environment to meet new people, which can also be very healthy.

If farmers' markets are not your thing, more and more shops are sourcing products from organic suppliers and supporting local and green initiatives. Nowadays, these choices are becoming more accessible, affordable, and easier to find.

On another side, having too many choices can become confusing. You can follow the guidelines in this book and try to simplify your shopping list. The simpler it is, the more likely you will maintain it in the long term.

Ultimately, caring for your well-being involves looking after each part that makes up your body and everything else you are part of—because you also depend on that.

6.7. The trend of sustainability: Why it is also for you

Sustainability today refers to the capacity to live within the planet's resources without damaging the environment. It is the key driver for innovation, but beyond that, it also means switching from self-centered attitudes to more unselfish mindsets.

Other newer terms like "regenerative" can be applied to agriculture, dietary approaches, or lifestyles. It refers to practices that help regrow or renew without depleting the earth.

What does a sustainable or regenerative diet look like for your health and the environment? It includes more plant-based foods, more nutrient-dense foods that prevent deficiencies, less waste, less sugar, fewer ultra-processed products, and less treating foods as objects to over-consume or as a distraction. This is not supposed to be a fashion or an imposition, because it is good for you and will make you happier.

Giving care to your health and well-being is not selfish and is your first responsibility. Caring too much about other things neglecting yourself can be an escape.

6.8. Tips to be healthy and eco-friendly

Here are some tips and ideas for taking care of yourself, your environment, and others. Keep it practical, simple, and easy without spending too much or adding unnecessary stress. Remember, it's better to start with a few simple changes and maintain them in the long-term rather than making too many changes at once and giving up soon after.

‣ Awareness

Awareness will help you become more present and understand yourself and life better, allowing you to see things more clearly. Take a moment to question the "why" of things and free yourself from unnecessary obligations or items. Stop and ask yourself if you really need to eat that, buy this, or go there. The relationship with yourself is the most important of all relationships.

‣ Make conscious choices

Observe the reason for your choices and their impact afterwards. Question the origin and content of what you consume, both physically and mentally.

‣ Be kind to people

Respect everyone and be kind to people because they have their own reasons and stories. Judgmental thoughts are like seeds against yourself and your health. There can't be real health without mental health, resentment, or excessive anger.

‣ Stay active

Find ways to move a little more every day, such as walking in parks, joining a sports club, doing outdoor workouts, going to the gym, cycling in your city, or taking the stairs.

‣ Consume less and reduce waste

Consume less of almost everything, reduce your waste, and start creating instead of only being a consumer. Support businesses and projects that promote this principle too.

‣ Keep it simple and think long-term.

Simplifying life a little bit is often a great way to become healthier and happier in the long term.

Last Thoughts

Don't do it all; just do your best

Please don't try to do everything at once; that is the best way to do nothing at all in the end. Going slowly, consistently, and patiently will certainly take you further.

Don't need to make changes if the timing isn't right. Keep it in your mind, and it will come to you when ready and needed. Consider it as an ongoing journey and focus on the long term, but don't accept feeling unwell as a normal state.

There are always ways to improve your quality of life, and it's definitely worth the effort. Physical challenges can also lead to significant transformations and personal evolution. So, keep investigating and exploring until you discover the root causes or change your perspective on life.

In the meantime, nurture yourself mentally by adding positive information, valuable knowledge, and inspiring reflections to your resources, including about health and holistic well-being.

And, remember this quote:

> "Do the best you can until you know better,
> then when you know better, do better" — Maya Angelou

Food Wisdom Series

Food Wisdom is a series of practical educational guides to learning about holistic health and nutrition in simple and accessible ways. Other titles available are:

The Energy & Habits Challenge

A 10-day plan to learn how to boost and maintain energy levels while adopting wholesome and healthy long-term habits. You will get the principles to apply, sample menus, and options to tailor the plan to fit popular diets, and tools to help you implement all this into your daily routine.

Foods for Your Brain & Emotions

A guide to understanding how food affects your brain, feeling, emotional states, and mental abilities. The boy has needs, as do the brain and nervous system, which mus be met to function properly. You will also find practical applications, mind-body techniques, and reflections about creating new long-term habits.

Consider this book just as a guide
to help you improve your choices
and become more aware of how they
impact your overall well-being.

However, do not use it as a tool to feed
your worries, you don't need more of them.
Your mental well-being is absolutely essential for
your health, and over-worrying will only hold you
back in life.

Allow yourself to be flexible and go with the flow,
slowly adapting more to your natural rhythm,
 and setting the conditions for your body to thrive.